Your Free Gift

I wanted to show my appreciation that you support my work so I've put together a free gift for you.

DISCOUNT, MUSIC FOR WORKOUTS, HEALTH CHECK-LIST

Visit the website http://www.motivy-fitness.com/

Just visit the link above to download it now.

I know you will love this gift.

Thanks!

Bruce Cleveland

I0408426

Table of Contents

ABOUT THE AUTHOR

Hello, my best friend. My name is Bruce Cleveland and I am happy, that you take the book, which i have written, in your hands.

Tell something about myself in order you realize why I decided to write a book. I am the professional sportman. At the age of 4 the parents decided that I am an active boy , brought me to the sport gimnastics, where I successfully was spending 20 years of my life.

I was the champion of my country and took part in the majority of international competitions. But the most valuable thing is since childhood i began to realize the value of health and physical development, which added the advantage more than one time either on the sportgrounds or in ordinary life.

I got secondary and high physical education.

After the finish of sport career, without thnking twice, I appeared in the fitness industry, decided to become the trainer of group programs, spent all classic classes with the usage of different equipment. I got the common fondation of our customers due to the charisma and the thoughtful approach to the business.

But it wasn't the surprise that the aerobics made me boring so quickly and uncomfortable and I was engaged in the personal training. So to speak with great enthusiam. It was urgent to continue the study and learn all principles of fitness workout more deeply.

I finished the dozen of courses of professional advancement and learnt the majority of content.I remembered everything I had learnt in the institute yet.

And I felt once again that everything proceeds well.

And life brought the surprise again. I got the invitation for job in the best circus of the world Cirque Du Soleil in the show of Alegria, which I went around 44 countries of the world with, and was in more than 100 countries. I got acquianted with the great quantity of interesting people.

I was working as the artist but in order not to lose physical habits I train the colleagues and managers of the circus staff.

During the finish of the career, I decided to get back to fitness, and realized that I have to start writing, sharing the knowledge, secrets and emotion, which were received for that period of time.

Why is this book for you?

I am sure, my dear reader, that you are not indifferent to healthy lifestyle.

From year to year you don`t want to lose the powers and get new micro-injuries, which get your nerves and follow you.

- You like spending your free time in action.

- You like the massage and you don`t like wasting odd money for it as I do.

- You spend a lot of time at the computer and it influences the common day activity and health.

- You like learn something new.

If the listed above points are all about you, don`t lose your time and pass the next chapter of my book.

How should you work with the book?

The important thing to read and not to use in practice that what you have found out is worse than not to read at all. You lose your time and don`t change your life for best. But I am sure you are not such person, my friend. That`s why we are working with the book.

- ✓ We are reading about the symptom and the zone of effect.

- ✓ We are learning what we should do and in what way, make the notes to the daybook, how often we should do this complex and pass to the action.

- ✓ We do, do, do and get the result.

So let's start

Chapter 1

A few words about Massage Therapy Balls

The power to massage your own body with therapy balls is a gift that keeps on giving. Various massage techniques have been around for thousands of years as ways to treat everyday aches and pains as well as injuries. While most massage requires a second person to do the work for you, all you need with massage balls is yourself. This means you can massage yourself any time, and reap the benefits!

Massage is known to have many health benefits from physical to mental. It can improve circulation, soothe sore muscles, break up scar tissue, lessen headaches, ease anxiety and more. It is estimated that 50% of people in the world will deal with chronic pain at some point in their lives. Doctors recommend massage all of the time- but they are often just not affordable on a regular basis. To have the best effect, massage should be performed consistently to keep muscles limber, and treat and prevent injuries and other painful conditions. With the massage therapy balls, you only have to invest in the set once. The only other investment you make is your time and commitment to yourself!

There are several different types of massage balls you can choose from depending on your needs. In general they are made of plastic, are slightly soft, but firm enough so you can send a good amount of pressure into the targeted area. They may differ in hardness or softness. Some may have knobs or ridges built into them, but usually you want them to have a nice, smooth surface. Depending on the severity of your pain, you may have to start with a softer ball and work your way up to something more penetrating.

If you have a specific problem area, the massage ball can be used specifically to isolate that spot. When used accordingly, it is very similar to deep tissue massage depending on how much pressure you apply. You are in control, which is also not normally the case in other massage situations. Depending on how you situate the balls, you could recreate the sensation of a therapists elbow digging into you right where you need it. It should not be painful at any time. Using the massage balls can help you take your pain management, and life, into your own hands.

What health conditions can massage therapy balls benefit? Here is a list:

- Low back pain
- Whiplash
- Arthritis
- Fibromyalgia
- Muscle strains and sprains
- Migraines
- Anxiety
- Depression
- Insomnia
- Fatigue
- PMS

Self massage can help to reduce dependency on medications such as pain relievers and anti-inflammatories, which are known to have many side effects. There are no side effects to these techniques except for an increased sense of well being. Massage is known to calm the mind and promote a sense of inner peace, which is how it helps people with mental disorders in addition to its physical component. It releases endorphins, which are the feel-good brain chemicals.

Massage is also known to stimulate immunity by activating the lymphatic system, which helps to clear toxins out of the body. It can improve range of motion and flexibility of joints and muscles, which keeps the body mobile. Stress, the culprit of many diseases, can also be greatly reduced through some me-time with massage balls. You can become your own therapist!

You can use the massage therapy balls on almost any part of the body. It is important to use them properly so as not to harm yourself. When learning how to use them, it is best to start in a larger muscle rather than directly on a joint. This way you can learn how to apply pressure, direction, and movement. Eventually you can use the ball to massage your joints with care.

To perform massage with the therapy balls, place the ball in the targeted area and move your body around on the ball. You may do this laying down, seated, or standing at a wall. You can move the body side to side, up and down, or in circular motions. For deep penetration, you can hold the ball completely still on an area such as a trigger point. A trigger point is a tender spot within a muscle that may radiate, or refer, pain elsewhere in the body. For example, hip pain may be caused by a trigger point in the lower back. When you have the technique down, you can even use two balls at once on certain areas, such as the back.

Application of self massage with therapy balls is a form of myofascial release. The entire body is connected through a sheath of tissue called the fascia. It is made of elastin and collagen and helps maintain the whole body. When the body is stressed, it can cause fascial dysfunction, results in a buildup of tissues rather than elasticity.

Chapter 2

Where to Use the Therapy Balls?

Head and Neck

For anyone who deals with tension headaches, migraines, neck pain, or is recovering from whiplash, the massage therapy balls can be very useful to alleviate pain in the head and neck. The muscles at the base of the skull, called the occipital lobe, are often neglected and become very tight over time. Tension in the muscles can develop into what feels like knots, tender areas, and loss of range of motion.

Neck Exercise #1: Headaches and Jaw Pain

To relieve neck pain, try lying down on the floor. Start with one ball underneath the occipital lobe and make a small nodding motion back and forth. Then, go side to side. Relax your jaw as you perform this action. Remember, the goal is to release tension.

You can perform this exercise twice daily, once in the morning and once at night before bed. Do this every day if you have a flare up, then every other day after symptoms subside. If the spot is too tender, try once a day or every other day. Regular use, at least once a week, will prevent pain from returning.

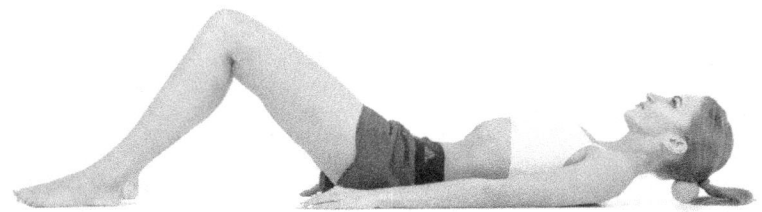

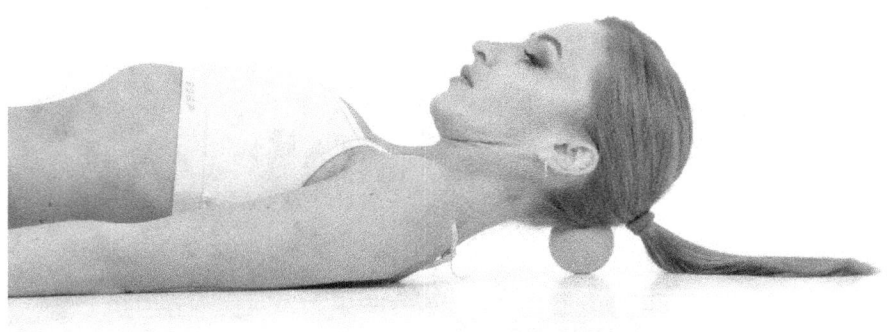

Neck Exercise #2: Cervical Spine Extensors

Grab your other ball and put them both in a sock or something to keep them close together. Lie back down, this time with the balls bracing either side or neck (not on the spine). Apply pressure on any tender spots in the neck. Hold in the area you need it and gently rock up and down to relieve tension and pain. To relieve pain and tension in the neck, you can even try targeting the upper back muscle the trapezius, where many trigger points often lie. Perform this once a day, or whenever you feel tension. The goal is to keep the muscles more relaxed from tensing up in the future.

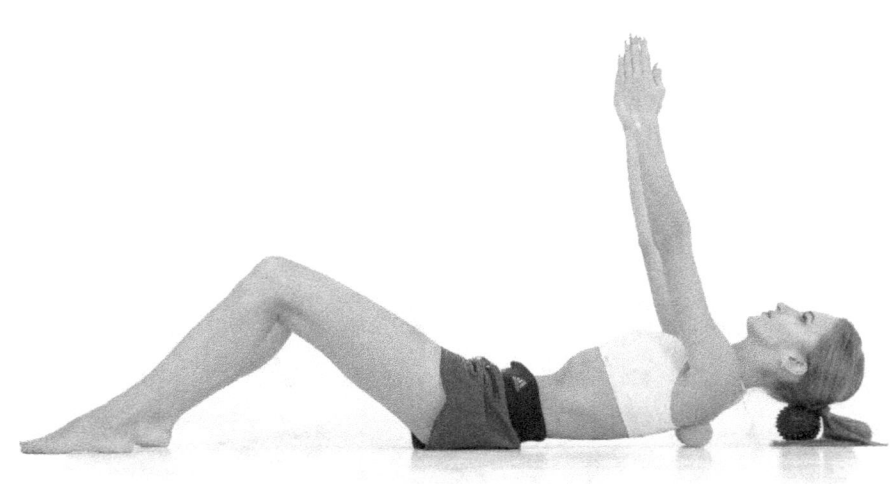

Neck Exercise #3: Whiplash

If you have pain at the front of your neck, which often contributes to a condition such as a 'forward head', you can try the balls on the front surface of the body. To do this, you must lie down on your belly and turn your head to one side. Place the ball under the inferior side and let it gently roll down. This part of the neck is very tender, so be careful with the pressure.

The main muscle targeted here is the sternocleidomastoid, however you can also roll out the scalenes, which attach the cervical vertebrae to the second rib. Both of these muscles often contribute to conditions such as whiplash, and when they are tightened, pull the head forward, out of proper alignment.

This exercise can be more intense, so it is recommended to do this once a day or every other day. Treating the front of the neck will help with muscular tightness that promotes poor posture (which often happens after whiplash), so the cervical spine can rest easier on the rest of the body.

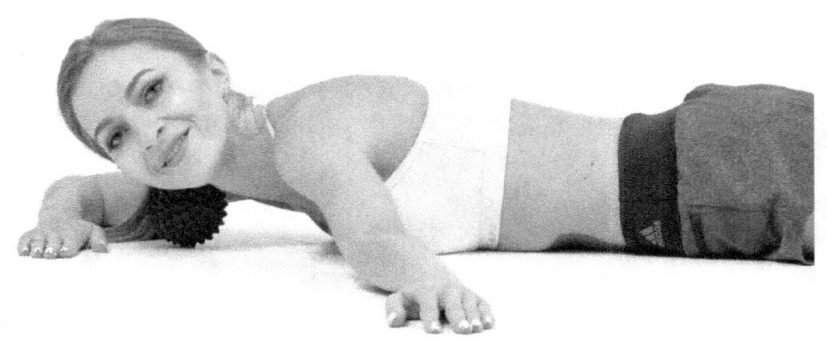

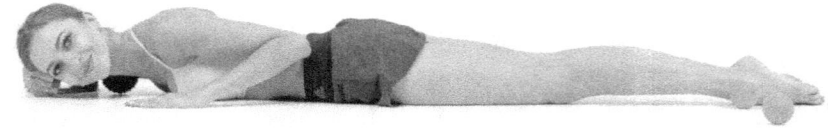

Upper Body

The upper body consists of the upper back, shoulders, and arms. There are many ways to use the massage balls for a variety of conditions affecting the upper body. These can include rotator cuff injuries, shoulder impingement syndrome, thoracic kyphosis, tendonitis, bursitis, tennis elbow, and carpal tunnel.

You can massage the shoulder joint either standing at a wall or reclined on the floor. Depending on your condition or pain may determine where you place the ball.

Upper Body Exercise #1: Impingement, Tendonitis, Bursitis

If you have any of these conditions, stand facing a wall and place the ball right in the center of the shoulder joint, where the humerus (upper arm bone) attaches to the rest of the shoulder. From there, make small circular motions in both directions. You can also roll the ball side to side to massage out the pectoralis (chest) muscle, which is often tight and down into the biceps tendon attachment and further down that muscle as well. You can also perform these lying down to give more pressure through using your body weight. It also requires a little balancing effort on your side as well. Do this exercise once per day with the goal of breaking up scar tissue and adhesions in the joint to promote better range of motion.

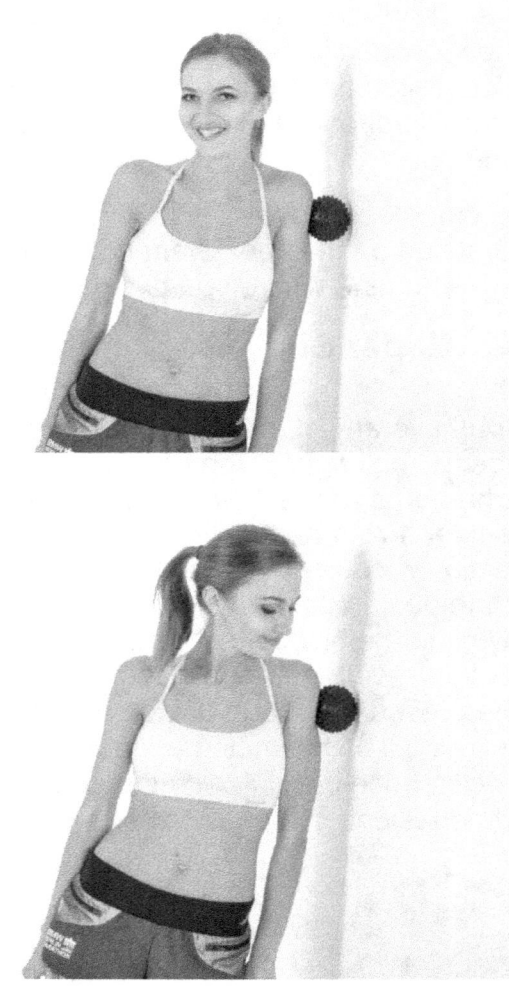

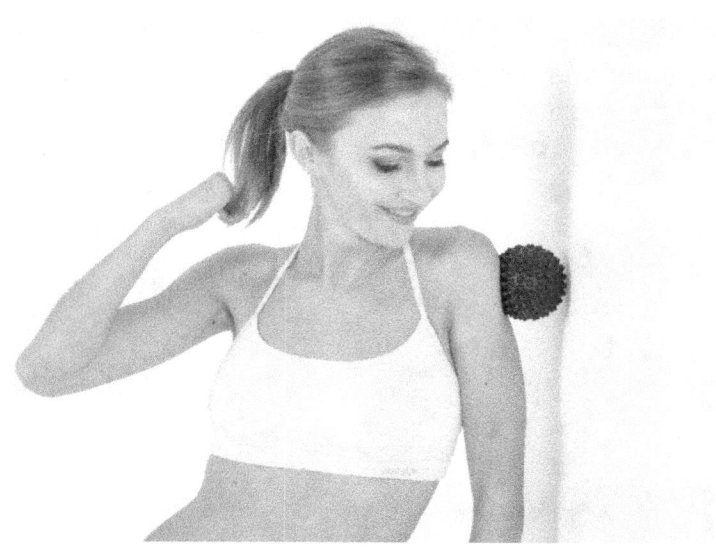

Upper Body Exercise #2: Deep Shoulder Trigger Points

There are also several trigger points deep inside the shoulder joint that are only accessible through the armpit. These muscles include the infraspinitis, subscapularis, teres minor, and teres major. Sometimes these trigger points can affect the surrounding areas, but in some cases they could even cause pain in the wrists similar to carpal tunnel syndrome. Using these massage techniques could possibly save you hundreds of dollars on doctors visits and unneeded x-rays if the problem never turned out to even really be carpal tunnel!

To get these pesky and hard to reach spots, again you can stand or lie down on your side. This time you will lift your arm up and place the ball in the area you need it- either a source of pain or a trigger point, while keeping the arm pressed into the wall. Try to roll it in the direction of the muscle if you can so that the ball does not slip away. For the standing variation, you must keep a very direct pressure between yourself and the wall so that it doesn't fall. Reaching higher points in the armpit may be more challenging and the reclined version may be better suited for that area.

It is recommended to do this once per day for painful, acute conditions and then every other day once initial pain subsides. Keep the muscles, joints, and fascia smooth here through regular use to prevent trigger points from returning.

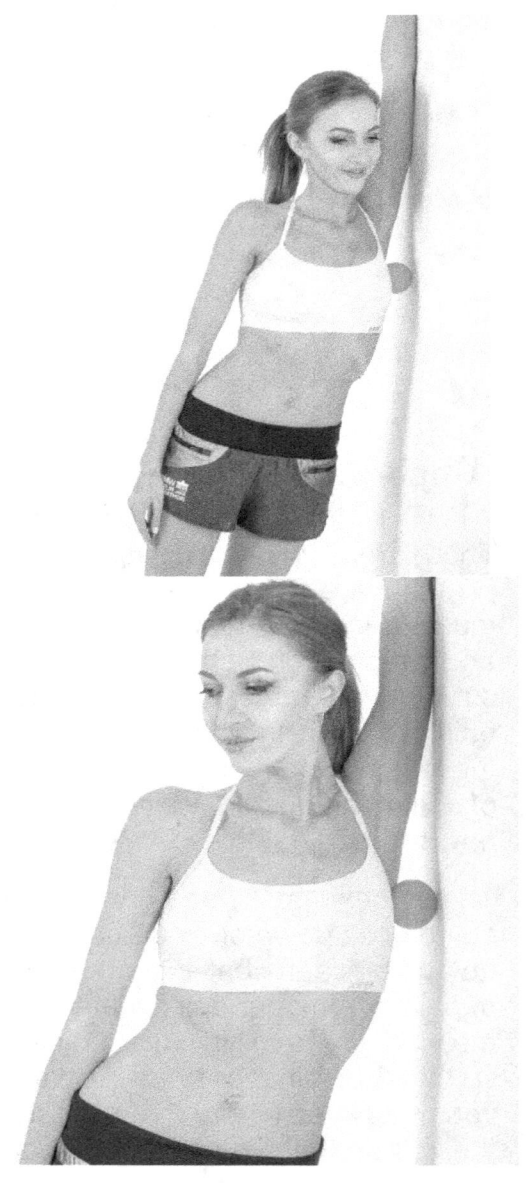

Upper Body Exercise #3: Tennis Elbow

Although called Tennis Elbow, pain in the elbow can occur from a number of things such as baseball pitching to golfing. Often the pain is referred from surrounding muscles in the forearm, specifically the extensor carpi radialis longus and the extensor digitorum muscles.

To get to these muscles, stand at the wall. Place the ball between the posterior (back of hand side) forearm and the wall. The extensor carpi radialis longus is located more to the inside of the arm, so you will have to rotate inward slightly to find the tender points to roll out. The extensor digitorums is more in the middle so it is easier to find. You will probably find the trigger points closer to the elbow, which is normal. Once you find a point, hold the ball on it for 5-30 seconds and repeat as often as needed.

This exercise should be done twice daily for initial symptoms, then once daily after a week, and eventually every other day. The goal is to relieve muscular tension around the elbow to promote full range of motion for various sports and activities.

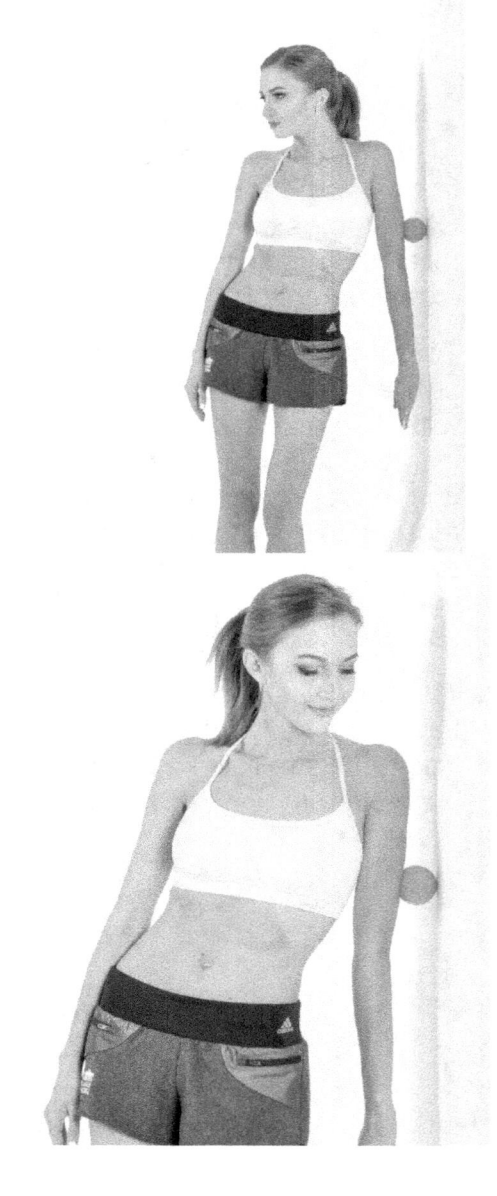

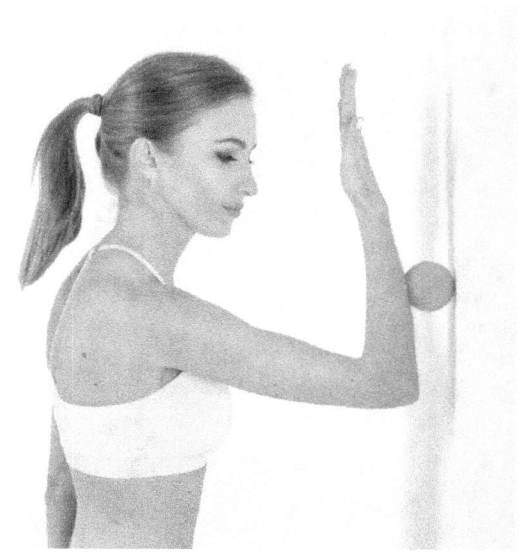

Upper Body Exercise #4: Carpal Tunnel Syndrome and Hand Pain

Carpal Tunnel Syndrome is only one of many issues that can affect the wrists and hands. If you work on a computer or play musical instruments professionally, hand and finger pain can be very real. To ease this pain and promote mobility, there may be several areas in the forearms that need massaged. These muscles include the

Take a seat at a table you can lean slightly into. Place one ball or two between the underside of your forearm and the table. These are the flexor muscles of the wrist and hand. Roll the ball(s) along the length of the muscle until your find a tender spot. Hold that area for as long as is comfortable.

Other areas that are well known to radiate pain, as well as numbness and tingling into the hands are the scalenes and other areas of the shoulder. This is because the trigger points that develop in those areas begin to compress nerves that run all the way down to the hands. So if the pain does not subside through initial treatment of the forearm, move up to your shoulder for secondary points.

You can perform massage on these areas twice a day to relieve pain in the wrists and hands.

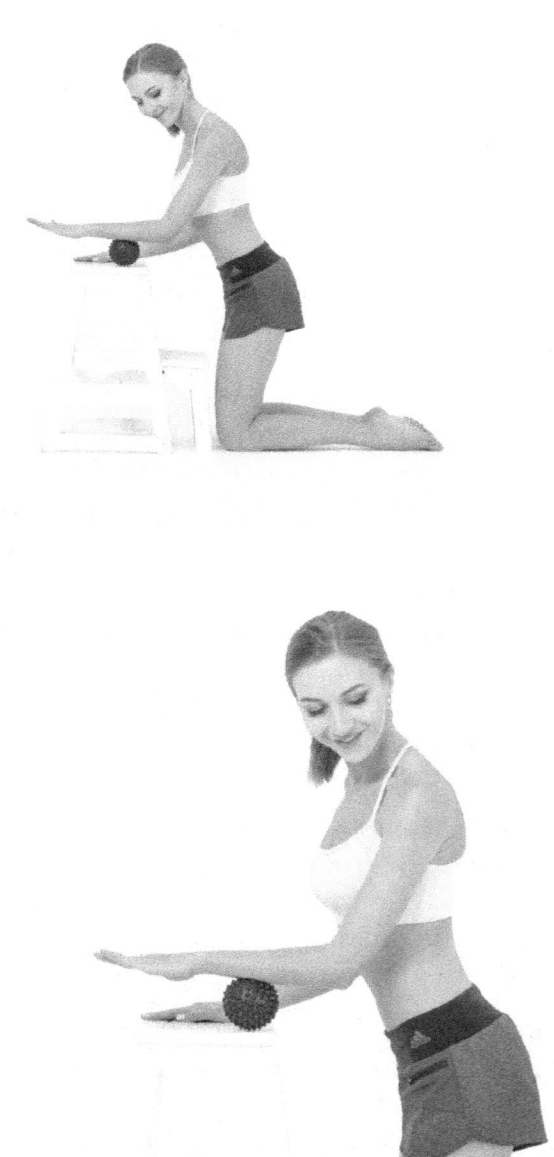

Upper Body Exercise # 5 Upper Back/Shoulder Pain

One of the best things you can do for yourself is to take both of your massage balls and slip them in a sock. Then place them between your shoulder blades on either side of your spine and invite sweet release into your body. This exercise targets the rhomboids, which are deeper muscles of the upper back that attach right under the scapula (shoulder blades), as well as the trapezius (large back muscle). Every felt like there is a spot under your shoulder that aches? This is the perfect solution.

You can do this lying on the floor or standing at a wall. Roll the balls up and down, or find a sweet spot and hold for 30 seconds. This is provides excellent stress relief, physically and mentally! You can do this one every day.

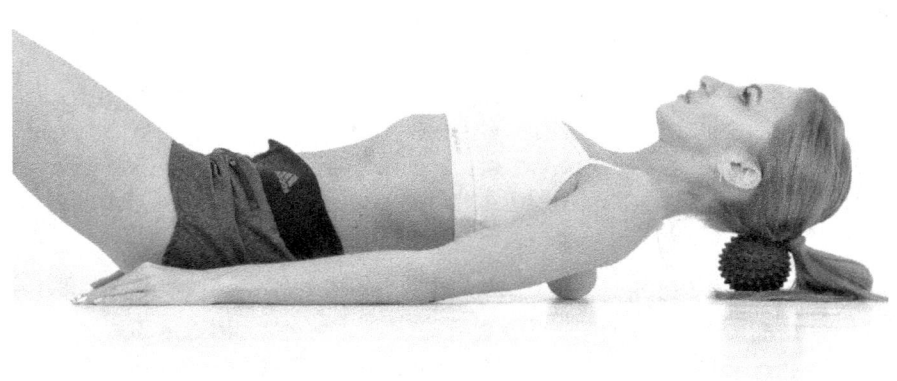

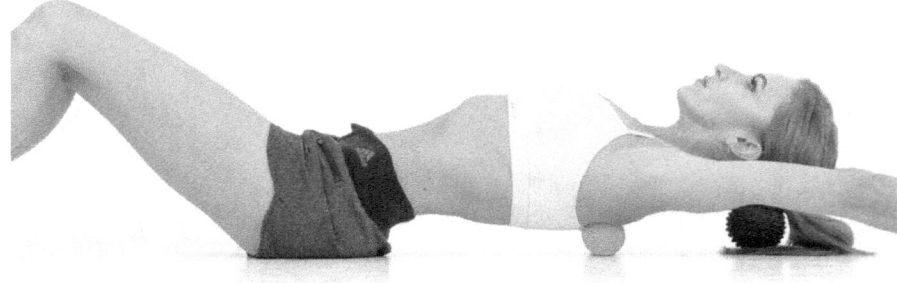

Lower Back + Hips

The lower back and hips are closely related when it comes to several pain and postural management issues here. The massage therapy balls can be helped to alleviate a number of conditions, from back pain due to an accident, postural imbalance, or spinal degeneration. These exercises are best done lying down on the back or the side.

Lower Back + Hips Exercise # 1

This one will be similar to the previous one, but instead you will do it for the lower back. Place the two balls in a sock and recline over them, one on either side of the spine. Start right below the rib cage and roll all the way down to your sacrum. There is a fascial band over the sacrum that often gets tights and can radiate pain along the low back and even the hips. If it hurts to roll the balls over the bones, either start with a softer ball or avoid going all the way down. When you find a specific area, you can rock back and forth or hold for 30 seconds.

Conversely, if the area of interest is a single spot further away from your spine, try reclining over just one ball and holding it there. You can do this one twice per day for initial symptoms, then gradually less as they fade. However, keep it up once per week to prevent pain from reoccurring.

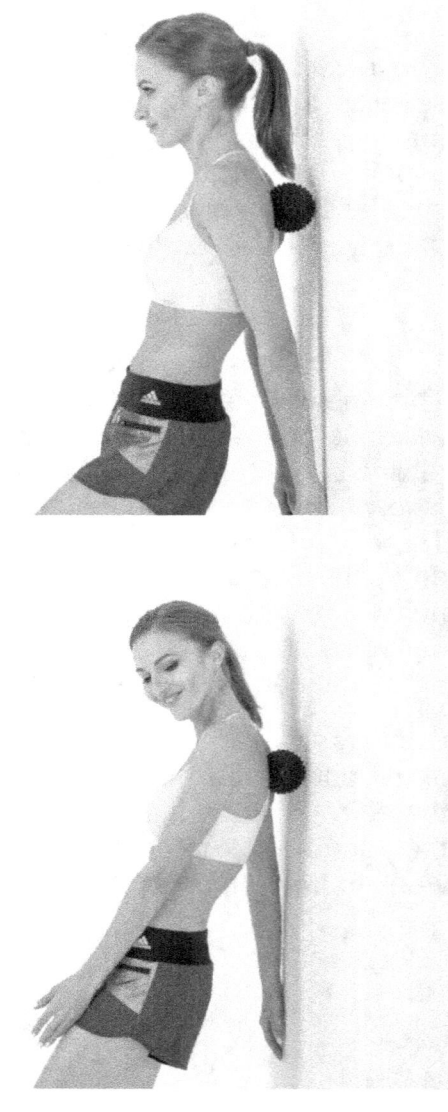

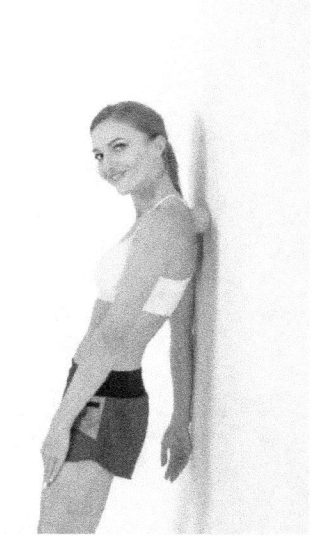

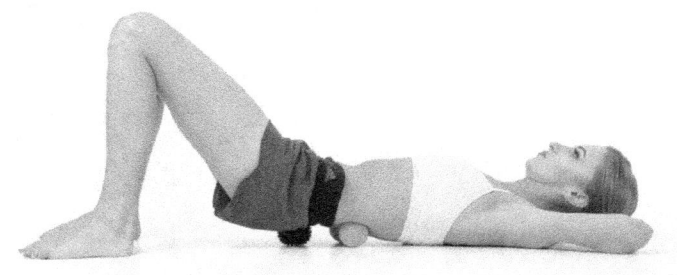

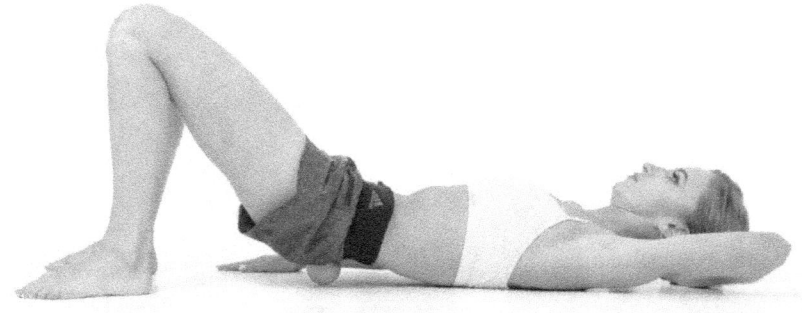

Lower Back + Hips Exercise #2: Sciatica + Piriformis Syndrome

Sciatica is a painful condition that originates in the lumbar vertebrae (lower back). It is a condition where the sciatic nerve becomes compressed and can cause pain, numbness, and tingling to radiate down the hip and even the entire leg. The root cause can vary, but it is generally thought to originate from misalignment or herniated discs in the lumbar spine.

Piriformis syndrome is sometimes related to sciatica, as when this muscle gets irritated, it can put pressure on the sciatic nerve. The piriformis is a deep gluteal muscle and attaches to the outer hip. It can spasm when overly tight or overworked and become painful and even tender.

To relieve symptoms of both these conditions, place the ball under the affected side by sitting on it. Roll the ball around until you find the tender area. It may be more to the side, in which case you will have to lean over and support yourself more with your arms. Hold the ball in place for 30 seconds, or try rolling it gently in circles. If the area is particularly tender, ease of the pressure by not leaning into it as much.

This exercise will help break up inflammation causing a painful piriformis and alleviate symptoms of sciatica. You can do this one daily.

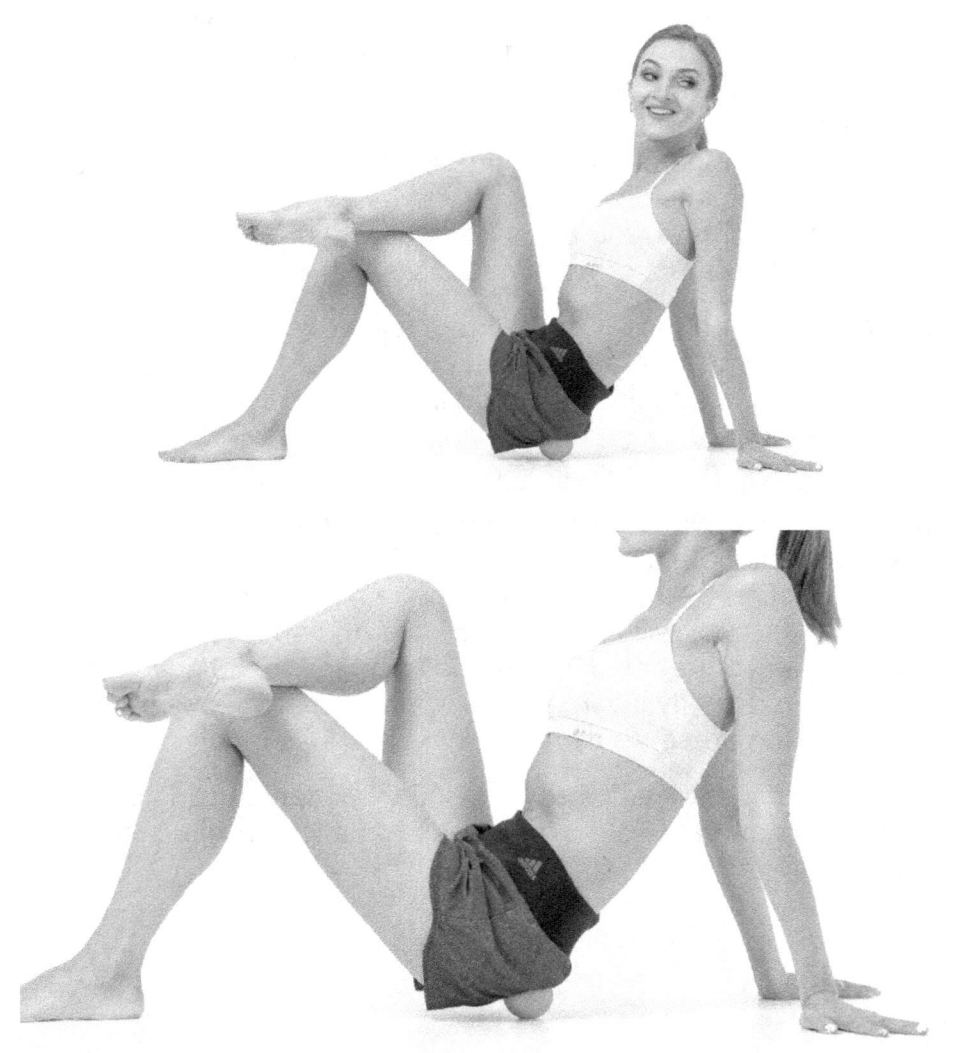

Lower Back + Hips Exercise #3 Correcting Pelvic Tilt

Pelvic tilt is an issue that effects the lumbar spine and moves the body out of neutral alignment. The two types of pelvic tilts are called posterior pelvic tilt and anterior pelvic tilt. A posterior pelvic tilt is when the pelvis tucks forward, which causes a tight lower back and tight hamstrings. Anterior pelvic tilt is when the hips point backward, decreasing the angle of the hips in front. This condition causes swayback, low back pain, and tight hip flexors.

To alleviate symptoms of these conditions, you can place the massage balls under your hamstrings or your hip flexors. Releasing these muscles will also help to correct the postural imbalances, too.

For issues with the posterior pelvic tilt, place the ball under your hamstring attachment, close to the hip joint. Place careful pressure on it and be mindful of your sitting bones. Hold the ball on any areas that feel tender, and then gently roll it down the entire length of the leg. The hamstring is actually made of three muscles, so be sure to also try the width of the leg as well.

If the problem is an anterior pelvic tilt, place the ball in your groin, where the hip flexors lie. This can be uncomfortable if you have never massaged this area before. The muscles are small and sensitive. Gently roll the ball forward and back to warm up the muscles. Then, hold in a specific spot that needs to be released for as long as is comfortable.

Pelvic tilt issues can seriously affect the quality of life because they do pull the spine out of alignment. If these issues are present, it is recommended to perform these twice per day in the beginning. Eventually you can decrease the amount of time as the symptoms and conditions relieve themselves. The goal is to not only relieve pain, but also to fix the underlying problems of alignment.

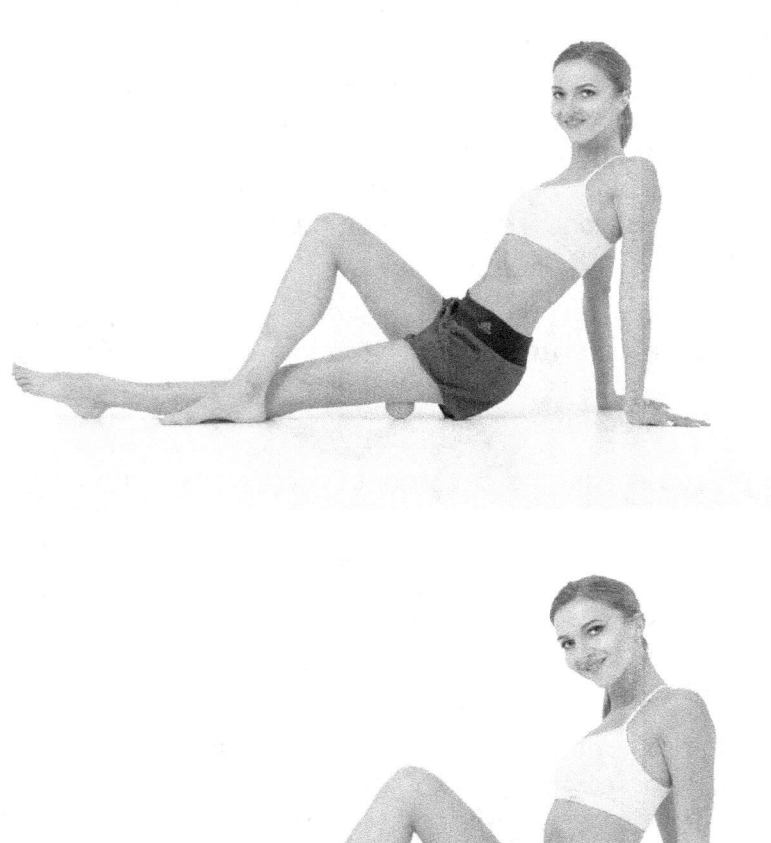

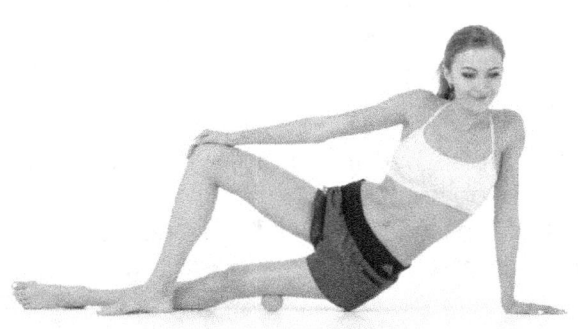

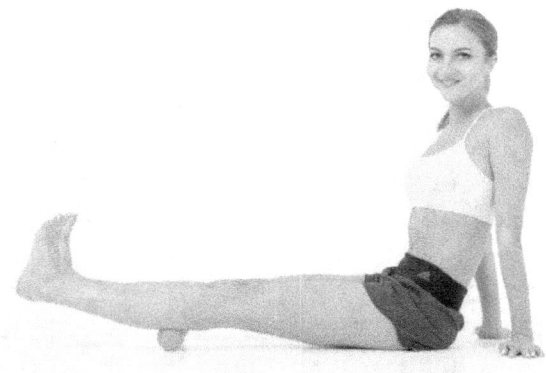

Lower Body Exercise #1: Plantar Fasciitis

Plantar Fasciitis is a condition affecting the bottom of the foot and most often manifests as heel pain. The plantar fascia runs the entire length of the bottom foot, from the heel, and becomes inflamed. The muscles surrounding the foot are tight and pull on the band of fascia. It is often most painful with walking or standing, and can feel like a sharp pain upon sudden movement.

Tight muscles around your feet pose risk for more serious injury, such as Achilles' tendon rupture. Often this condition may also occur due to the bones shifting in the feet. This happens when the natural arch of the foot begins to collapse. This could happen for several reasons, such as overuse, improper footwear, or misalignment over the years wearing down the bones and joints.

One of the most effective remedies for immediate pain relief is to stand on the massage therapy ball. Place it right underneath the tender spot and hold it there for 30 seconds to 1 minute. You can also do this seated at a desk, and apply less pressure.

You also want to target your calves with the balls for plantar fasciitis as well. Take a seat and place the ball right under you knee, in the meat of the calf muscle (not in the crease of the knee joint itself). Roll it down toward the Achilles and notice any trigger points. Hold those areas. This will help loosen the muscles so that not only provides pain relief but also can help alleviate the condition. Do these daily for acute symptoms and then work into your routine weekly after the condition subsides to prevent it from returning.

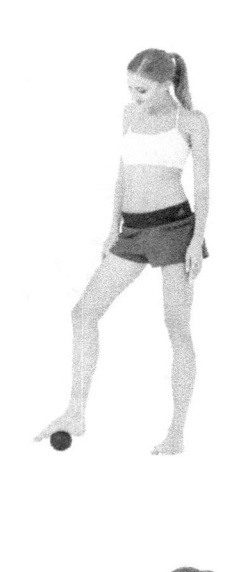

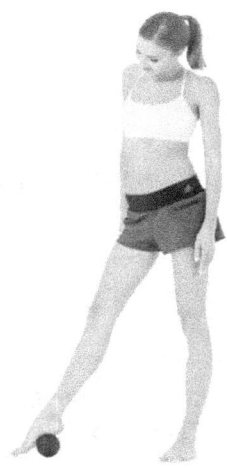

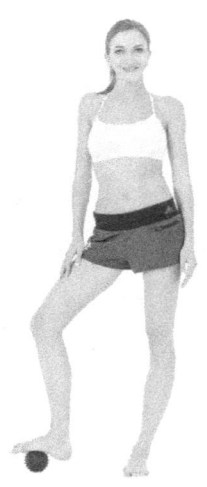

Conclusion

Incorporating massage therapy balls into your health and self-care regimen has numerous benefits for a variety of conditions. Whether you are looking to treat or prevent a muscular or postural injury, self-massage through this targeted therapy can increase blood flow, decrease pain, and improve overall well-being. It takes some dedication, but with regular practice, the results will be immense improvement for whatever condition you are seeking to treat.

Chapter 3

A parting word

Well done, my reader!

You have worked through this small handbook of the improvement of the life quality, whereas other people don`t care about it. The small thing is left to do is to develop the everyday habit of exercises with massage balls and common physical training and from year to year you become more perfect. It is obvious you have also the same goal as mine to live till 100 years and herewith to be absolutely active and adequate-thinking person.

That`s why you don`t give up and I believe in you.

In order to your life is full and pain and illnesses don`t make you crazy , we made the small and very sufficient checklist. You find 4 important points there. Not finishing off even one of them means no to become superman.

These points are following:

- **Training**

We as any device requires the charging. The telephone is charging due to the power socket, and we are charging due to physical exercises and making all our systems in action.

- **Nutrition**

As for any car , the oil for our organism is the refill of nutrients. We can refill ourselves with second quality oil and in inadequate quantity. But we can treat it seriously and with full responsibilty and change our habits of nutrition for best.

- **The drinking schedule**

We consists of water in many percents; muscles, bones, eyes, brains have more more quantity of water. What happens if we stop providing the water to our organism. Sure, it becomes worse. That`s why you should treat this drinking schedule seriously.

- **Sleep**

During the sleep we are growing. As our mothers have said in the childhood in such way and they were right. During the sleep we are recovering, growing, healing up the wounds and rest morally. Don`t take away the rest for your organism and it gives you productivity and vigorous health.

After signing up, you can find the test for understanding your starting point and simple sufficient chacklist, which makes you a **superman.**

Your Free Gift

I wanted to show my appreciation that you support my work so I've put together a free gift for you.

DISCOUNT, MUSIC FOR WORKOUTS, HEALTH CHECK-LIST

Visit the website http://www.motivy-fitness.com/

Just visit the link above to download it now.

I know you will love this gift.

Thanks!

Bruce Cleveland